Exposures to Lead and Other Metals at an Aircraft Repair and Flight School Facility

Lilia Chen, MS, CIH
Judith Eisenberg, MD, MS

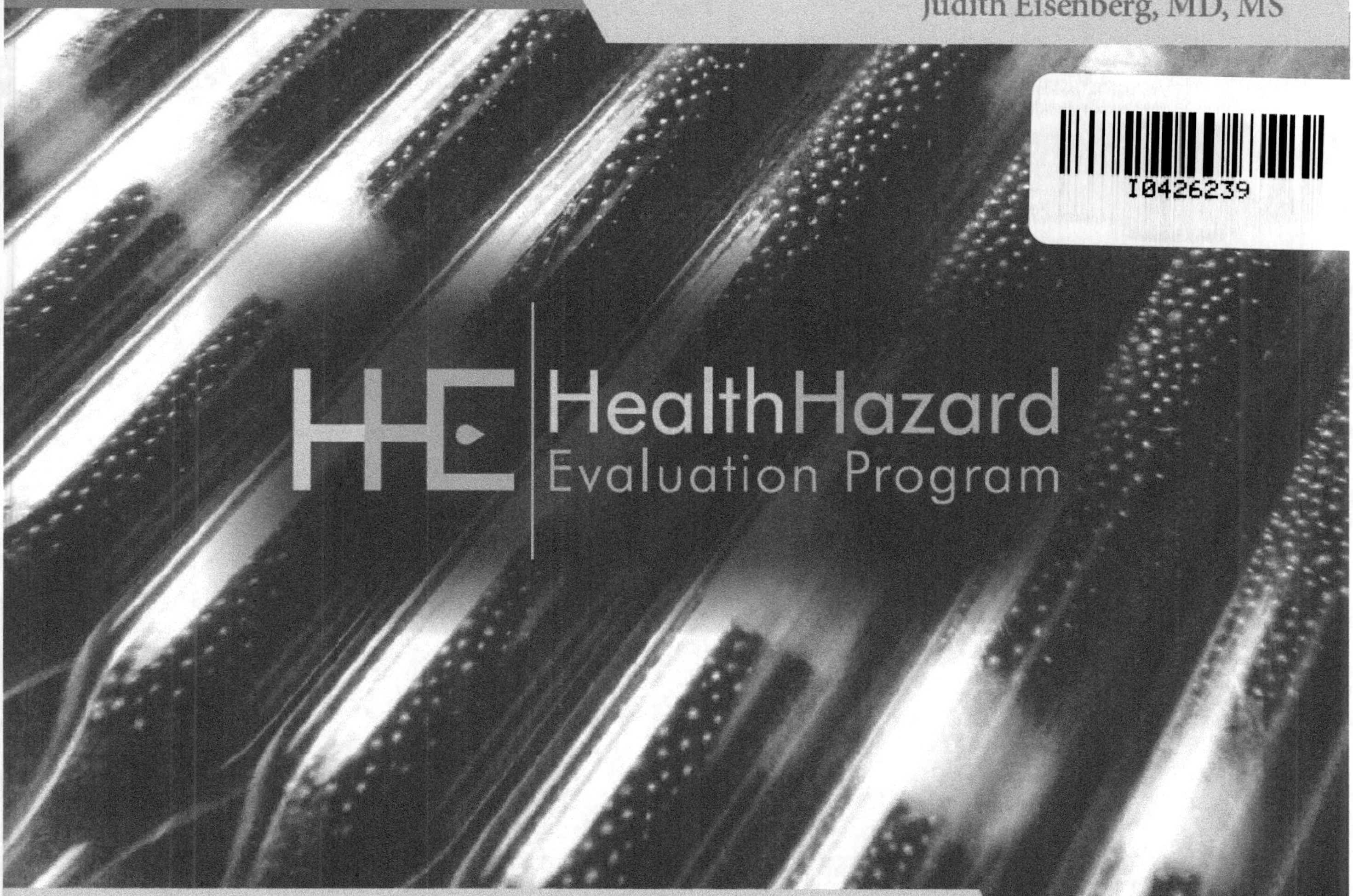

HHE HealthHazard Evaluation Program

Report No. 2012-0115-3186
July 2013

U.S. Department of Health and Human Services
Centers for Disease Control and Prevention
National Institute for Occupational Safety and Health

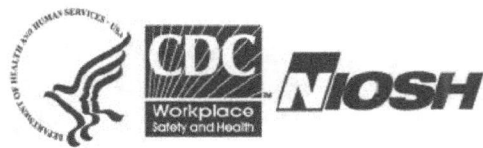

Contents

The employer is required to post a copy of this report for 30 days at or near the workplace(s) of affected employees. The employer must take steps to ensure that the posted report is not altered, defaced, or covered by other material.

The cover photo is a close-up image of sorbent tubes, which are used by the HHE Program to measure airborne exposures. This photo is an artistic representation that may not be related to this Health Hazard Evaluation.

Highlights of this Evaluation

The Health Hazard Evaluation Program received a request from the owners of an aircraft repair and flight school facility. The owners submitted the request because of concerns about lead exposure. The single-engine aircrafts use leaded aviation fuel, which generates lead-containing dust as a combustion byproduct.

What We Did

- We visited the facility in May 2012.
- We interviewed the owners and employees about their health, job duties, previous blood lead testing, and personal protective equipment use.
- We collected blood samples to check lead levels.
- We collected air samples for elements, including inorganic and organic lead.
- We collected surface wipe samples for lead throughout the workplace, from employees' hands, and inside employees' personal vehicles.
- We reviewed the labeling and storage of chemicals.
- We observed and asked about housekeeping and personal protective equipment use.

What We Found

- No one reported symptoms related to their work.
- All airborne concentrations of lead and other elements measured over a work shift were low.
- Lead was detected in the blood of all facility personnel.
- The airborne lead concentration during sandblasting of spark plugs approached an occupational exposure limit for a short-term exposure.
- The hangar area had the highest surface concentrations of lead.
- Lead was found on the steering wheel of an employee's car.
- Lead dust was found on toys and a baby walker in work areas.
- Chemicals were improperly labeled and stored.
- There was no schedule for regular cleaning of the hangar, and a leaf blower was reportedly used to clear dust from surfaces.
- Employees prepared and stored food near the aircraft repair area.

> We were asked to evaluate the workplace for lead exposures after all employees and a minor child who was often present at the facility were found to have detectable blood lead levels. Air and surface wipe samples confirmed the presence of lead in the workplace. Airborne personal breathing zone sample concentrations were below occupational exposure limits. Our testing confirmed the previous blood lead results. We recommended administrative controls to further reduce lead exposures in the workplace and keep lead from leaving the workplace. Children should not be allowed in a workplace that would place them at risk for exposure to lead and other health and safety hazards.

What We Found (continued)

- Small parts, tools, and metal shavings on and around the workbench area, desktops, and open shelving units posed a safety hazard.

What the Employer Can Do

- Require respirator use during sandblasting of spark plugs. Develop a respiratory protection program as required by the Occupational Safety and Health Administration.

- Store chemicals in labeled, closed containers, within safety cabinets.

- Avoid dry cleaning methods, such as a leaf-blower, or dry sweeping. Use wet cleaning methods instead as part of a regular cleaning schedule.

- Move food preparation and storage areas out of the hangar. Do not allow eating, drinking, or smoking inside the hangar area.

- Have employees wash hands before eating to prevent ingestion of lead-containing dust.

- Provide disposable shoe covers and on-site laundering of work clothes to reduce the potential for take-home lead contamination.

- Do not allow children in the work areas.

What Employees Can Do

- Wear a respirator when sandblasting spark plugs.

- Do not eat or drink in the hangar area.

- Wash hands thoroughly before eating and drinking, before and after putting on gloves, and before leaving the workplace.

- Leave work clothes at the workplace.

- Wear disposable shoe covers when working, and throw them away before leaving work.

- Cover and label all containers of waste chemicals, such as drained engine oil.

Mention of any company or product does not constitute endorsement by NIOSH. In addition, citations to websites external to NIOSH do not constitute NIOSH endorsement of the sponsoring organizations or their programs or products. Furthermore, NIOSH is not responsible for the content of these websites. All web addresses referenced in this document were accessible as of the publication date of this report.

Abbreviations

$\mu g/4$ inches^2	Micrograms per 4 square inches
$\mu g/dL$	Micrograms per deciliter
$\mu g/m^3$	Micrograms per cubic meter
ACGIH®	American Conference of Governmental Industrial Hygienists
AL	Action level
BLL	Blood lead level
CFR	Code of Federal Regulations
EPA	Environmental Protection Agency
MDC	Minimum detectable concentration
MQC	Minimum quantifiable concentration
NAICS	North American Industry Classification System
NIOSH	National Institute for Occupational Safety and Health
OEL	Occupational exposure limit
OSHA	Occupational Safety and Health Administration
ppm	Parts per million
PEL	Permissible exposure limit
REL	Recommended exposure limit
STEL	Short-term exposure limit
TEL	Tetraethyl lead
TLV®	Threshold limit value
TWA	Time-weighted average
WEEL™	Workplace environmental exposure level

Introduction

In March 2012, the Health Hazard Evaluation Program received a request from the owners of an aircraft repair and flight school facility in Colorado to evaluate employee lead exposures. This was in response to concerns about lead exposure which began when a child who was at the worksite nearly every day was found to have a blood lead level (BLL) above 10 micrograms per deciliter (μg/dL); the CDC "level of concern" at the time of the site visit [CDC 1991]. The owners and employees were subsequently tested and found to have had BLLs less than 10 μg/dL; the National Institute for Occupational Safety and Health (NIOSH) adult blood lead reference value. The NIOSH Adult Blood Lead Epidemiology and Surveillance (ABLES) program tracks elevated BLLs (i.e. BLLs at or above the reference value) among adults in the U.S. [CDC 2011].

We visited the facility in May 2012. We held an opening meeting with the owners and employees, a family doctor who provided care for the family with the elevated lead level, and a representative from the U.S. Environmental Protection Agency (EPA) Region 8. Afterwards, we toured the work and office areas.

Because of the child's elevated BLL, the EPA representative tested the family's home to assess non-occupational sources of lead exposure. We provided contact information for experts in pediatric lead poisoning to the family doctor. Educational documents regarding pediatric lead poisoning [CDC 2009] were distributed at the closing meeting. An interim letter with results and preliminary recommendations was provided in August 2012 and, in September 2012, the owners and employees were sent their individual blood lead test results.

The facility offered aircraft maintenance and rental services and flight instruction for pilot certificates. The owners and two employees worked at the facility. The owners split their time between this facility and a second facility in another state. One employee was a part-time flight instructor, and one employee was a mechanic who worked in the hangar 40 hours or more a week. The facility was a single story aircraft hangar with walls made from unpainted concrete slabs, and a concrete floor painted with yellow lines. A shop area with workbenches and tools was on the south side of the hangar. Metal storage cabinets lined part of the south side and most of the west side of the hangar. These cabinets contained supplies for aircraft maintenance and repair, including solvents and paints. The east side of the hangar was separated from the rest of the building by drywall, creating a two-level office space. The first floor had a reception area with a retail counter, restroom, and waiting area, and the second floor had a carpeted classroom, carpeted office, and storage area. The storage area had no drywall ceiling and was open to the hangar area.

Aircraft at this facility used Avgas 100LL fuel, which contains an organic form of lead called tetraethyl lead (TEL). According to the Avgas manufacturer's analysis (Delek Refining), the amount of TEL in the two batches of Avgas 100LL fuel delivered prior to our visit ranged from 1.75 to 1.84 grams of lead per gallon. Aircraft were fueled from a tanker truck outside of the hangar.

The use and maintenance of aircraft fueled with leaded gasoline creates a risk of lead exposure for employees working in and around these vehicles. When leaded aviation fuel is burned in an aircraft's engine, about 95% of the lead is expelled from the combustion chamber as elemental/inorganic lead dust; while 5% of the lead is retained inside the engine and the engine oil [EPA 2008]. This lead-containing dust coats engine parts and other surfaces in and around the aircraft, especially areas exposed to the exhaust plume. Aircraft exhaust is well-recognized as a major contributor of lead pollution in the soil and air. A recent study found elevated BLLs in children living within 500 meters of an airport [Miranda et al. 2011]. EPA recently estimated that 16 million people live within one kilometer of the nearly 20,000 airport facilities in this country and that 3 million children attend a school located within the same one kilometer radius. The EPA estimates that aviation fuel accounts for half of the lead released into the air in this country. The EPA estimates that between 1970 and 2008, approximately 14.6 billion gallons of Avgas was used, resulting in the emission of about 34,000 tons of inorganic lead [EPA 2010]. A detailed discussion of lead and its health effects can be found in the appendix.

Methods

We interviewed the owners and employees about health issues they felt were related to their job, job duties, and personal protective equipment use. We also observed work practices and collected blood for BLLs and urine samples for TEL. Urine would be tested for TEL only if the BLL was above 10 µg/dL.

We collected five area air samples in the hangar and office areas and four full-shift personal breathing zone air samples for elements (minerals and metals) on mixed cellulose ester filters and TEL on XAD-2 tubes in series. The filters were analyzed using National Institute for Occupational Safety and Health (NIOSH) Method 7303 [NIOSH 2013]. The XAD-2 tubes were desorbed using n-pentane and analyzed using high performance liquid chromatography using a Bureau Veritas North America method. The minimum detectable concentrations (MDCs) and minimum quantifiable concentrations (MQCs) were calculated by dividing the analytical limits of detection and quantitation (mass units) by the minimum volume of air sampled. The MDCs and MQCs represent the smallest air concentrations that could have been detected (MDC) or quantified (MQC) for the volume of air sampled. We also collected a task-based air sample when an employee sandblasted spark plugs, and a short-term area air sample at the exhaust of a running aircraft engine for elements and TEL.

Surface wipe samples were collected in the hangar and adjacent offices using General Electric Healthcare Whatman™ smear filters moistened with isopropanol. The wipe samples were analyzed according to NIOSH Method 7303 [NIOSH 2013]. Hand wipe samples were collected with SKC Full Disclosure® Instant Wipes. After collection, each wipe was sprayed with a 5% leaching solution of acetic acid to solubilize lead and lead compounds into lead ions. The wipe was then sprayed with a chilled solution of sodium rhodizonate, a chemical that reacts colorimetrically to the presence of lead by changing from yellow to red. The visual limit of identification for the method is approximately 17–20 micrograms per sample.

The hand wipe samples were then analyzed for elements according to NIOSH Method 7303 [NIOSH 2013]. The wipe sample analyses identified lead ions and could not distinguish inorganic lead from TEL.

Results and Discussion

We interviewed the two owners and two employees, each of whom gave informed consent for blood and urine testing. Three were male, and one was female. They ranged in age from 31 to 63 years. All stated they performed aircraft fueling. None reported symptoms that they related to work. None of the BLLs were above 10 μg/dL [CDC 2011], so urine samples were not tested for organic lead.

All full-shift airborne concentrations of elements and TEL were below applicable occupational exposure limits (OELs) (Table 1). The highest personal breathing zone air concentration of inorganic lead was 3.5 micrograms per cubic meter (μg/m³), well below the Occupational Safety and Health Administration (OSHA) permissible exposure limit (PEL), NIOSH recommended exposure limit (REL), and American Conference of Governmental Industrial Hygienists (ACGIH) threshold limit value (TLV) of 50 μg/m³. The highest personal breathing zone air concentration measured for TEL was 8.3 μg/m³, below the

Table 1. Personal breathing zone air sampling results for inorganic and tetraethyl lead*

Job title	Pump time (minutes)	Volume (m³)	Analyte	Concentration (μg/m³)	MDC (μg/m³)	MQC (μg/m³)
Mechanic	559	0.551	Inorganic lead	3.5	0.54	1.8
			Tetraethyl lead	8.3†	0.16	2.2
Flight Instructor	262	0.258	Inorganic lead	ND‡	1.2	3.9
			Tetraethyl lead	6.2†	0.35	4.7
Manager	550	0.490§	Inorganic lead	ND	0.61	2.0
			Tetraethyl lead	[0.78]¶	0.18	2.4
Owner	526	0.481	Inorganic lead	ND	0.62	2.1
			Tetraethyl lead	[0.75]	0.19	2.5
OSHA PEL (8-hour TWA)			Inorganic lead	50		
NIOSH REL (8-hour TWA)			Inorganic lead	50		
OSHA PEL (8-hour TWA)			Tetraethyl lead	75		
NIOSH REL (up to 10-hour TWA)			Tetraethyl lead	75		

TWA = Time-weighted average

*Tetraethyl lead can be absorbed through the skin.

†Breakthrough of approximately 15% was observed on the back-up tube, thus the concentration may be underestimated.

‡Not detected

§Pump precalibration and postcalibration difference was 13%. The lower flow rate was used to calculate the concentration.

¶Concentrations between the MDC and MQC are shown in brackets to acknowledge that there is more uncertainty associated with these values than with concentrations above the MQC.

OSHA PEL and NIOSH REL of 75 µg/m³, and ACGIH TLV of 100 µg/m³. Other elements quantified in the personal breathing zone air samples included chromium, iron, titanium, and zinc. The concentrations of these metals are not included in the tables because they were all low, less than 10% of the most conservative OELs.

No inorganic lead was found in area air samples, and concentrations of TEL were low, between the MDC and MQC inside the hangar (Table 2). Other elements quantified in the area air samples in the hangar and offices included aluminum, chromium, copper, iron, manganese, strontium, and zinc. The concentrations of these metals are not included in the tables because they were very low (less than 5 µg/m³).

Table 2. Area air samples taken in the hangar for inorganic and tetraethyl lead*

Area	Pump time (minutes)	Volume (m³)	Analyte	Concentration (µg/m³)	MDC	MQC
					(µg/m³)	
South hangar next to work bench	564	0.562	Inorganic lead	ND†	0.54	1.8
			Tetraethyl lead	[1.4]‡	0.16	2.1
North hangar	564	0.532	Inorganic lead	ND	0.56	1.9
			Tetraethyl lead	[0.73]	0.17	2.3
Upstairs office on desk	388	0.388	Inorganic lead	ND	0.77	2.6
			Tetraethyl lead	[1.2]	0.23	3.1
Upstairs office at entryway floor level	542	0.537	Inorganic lead	ND	0.56	1.9
			Tetraethyl lead	[0.73]	0.17	2.2
Outside hangar	548	0.536	Inorganic lead	ND	0.56	1.9
			Tetraethyl lead	ND	0.17	2.2

*Tetraethyl lead can be absorbed through the skin.

†Not detected

‡Concentrations between the MDC and MQC are shown in brackets to acknowledge that there is more uncertainty associated with these values than with concentrations above the MQCs.

The task-based and short-term air sampling results are shown in Table 3. The concentration of inorganic lead was 219 µg/m³ on the employee sandblasting spark plugs for 12 minutes. The sandblaster was stored and used in a metal cabinet next to the work bench. The activity was performed on the sandblasting machine, which remained on the shelf in the cabinet while the employee stood in front of the open cabinet. There are no short-term exposure limits for inorganic lead; however, ACGIH recommends that under no circumstance should the exposure exceed five times the TLV-TWA (50 µg/m³ for inorganic lead) excursion limit of 250 µg/m³. Although this one sample (219 µg/m³) did not exceed the excursion limit, we cannot rule out the possibility that an exposure exceeding the excursion limit may occur.

Table 3. Task-based and short term air samples for inorganic and tetraethyl lead*

Area/Task	Pump time (minutes)	Volume (m³)	Analyte	Concentration (µg/m³)	MDC (µg/m³)	MQC (µg/m³)
Task based sample – sandblasting spark plugs	12	0.012	Inorganic lead	219	25	83
			Tetraethyl lead	ND†	7.5	100
Short term sample at airplane exhaust	15	0.015	Inorganic lead	ND	20	67
			Tetraethyl lead	ND	6	80

*Tetraethyl lead can be absorbed through the skin.

†Not detected

Surface wipe samples for elements were taken throughout the aircraft hangar and office areas. Quantifiable concentrations of aluminum, barium, cadmium, chromium, cobalt, copper, iron, lead, magnesium, manganese, molybdenum, nickel, strontium, tin, titanium, vanadium, and zinc were identified in the wipe samples. Few standards define "acceptable" levels of workplace surface contamination. Wipe samples, however, can provide information regarding the effectiveness of housekeeping practices, the potential for exposure to contaminants by skin absorption or ingestion (e.g., surface contamination on a table that is also used for food consumption), the potential for contamination of worker clothing and subsequent transport of the contaminant outside the workplace, and the potential for non-process related activities (e.g., sweeping) to generate airborne contaminants.

The results of lead levels from the surface wipe samples are provided in Table 4. The highest levels of lead were found in the hangar area on the painted yellow line (13 micrograms per 4 square inches [µg/4 inches²]) and on and around the work bench (6.5 to 12 µg/4 inches²). Lower amounts of lead were observed in the dust from the upstairs office (ND to 1.3 µg/4 inches²). The surface of the baby walker in the hangar also had a detectable level of inorganic lead (0.28 µg/4 inches²). A refrigerator, microwave, charcoal grill, and toaster oven were located in the hangar approximately 15 feet from the workbench, and employees reported eating and drinking in the hangar. It is possible for lead-containing dust to contaminate eating surfaces and food storage and cooking appliances.

Employees used a NIOSH-approved half-mask elastomeric respirator with organic vapor cartridges when spray painting. Although this activity was not performed during our evaluation, the employees who used this respirator reported never being fit tested or medically cleared for respirator use. The respirator was stored on the work bench, and the sample collected from the inside of the respirator had a quantifiable level of lead (0.28 µg/4 inches²).

Table 4. Surface wipe sample results for lead

Location	Lead level (μg/4 inches^2)
In the upstairs office:	
Top of heat vent near floor	1.3
Top of bookcase	0.63
Table surface	ND*
Bottom of bookcase near floor	ND
Desk in front of computer	ND
Hangar area:	
Floor – on painted yellow line	13
Floor in front of work bench	12
Top of workbench	6.5
Workbench in southwest corner	2.3
Floor under plane in middle of hangar	1.9
Middle step leading from hangar to office	1.1
Floor of hangar entry	0.85
Cardboard liner used as a mat	0.33
Baby walker	0.28
Top of cart	ND
Other areas:	
Golf cart seat	0.45
Inside respirator†	0.28
Table in waiting area	ND
Floor entering waiting area	ND
Door handle from hangar into office†	ND
Baby toy†	ND
Outside of hangar (sign surface)	ND
Inside plane on yoke†	ND
Inside owner's car – driver's seat	ND
MDC	0.08
MQC	0.21

*Not detected
†Approximate estimation of surface area

We collected wipe samples from the hands of two employees for quantitative analysis of elements (Table 5). Lead, cadmium, chromium, nickel, and zinc were found on the employees' hands after they ate lunch. The mechanic had levels of lead, cadmium, and zinc that exceeded 100 μg/sample after finishing the work shift but before washing his hands. The mechanic reported using latex or nitrile gloves most of the time when handling grease and oil.

Table 5. Hand wipe results for elements

Employee	Analyte	Level (μg/sample)
Employee's hands after lunch (reported no hand washing)	Lead	34
	Cadmium	5.8
	Chromium	1.2
	Nickel	1.3
	Zinc	45
Mechanic's hands after work (reported no hand washing)	Lead	530
	Cadmium	140
	Chromium	17
	Copper	41
	Zinc	150

Colorimetric wipe tests of two mechanics' hands done upon completion of routine work tasks indicated the presence of lead (Figure 1). A colorimetric wipe showed no lead on an employee's hands after hand washing. The employee reported washing his hands up to 10 times per day, sometimes using kerosene to remove engine grease. A colorimetric wipe used on the steering wheel of an employee's car showed lead contamination, indicating the potential for take-home exposure.

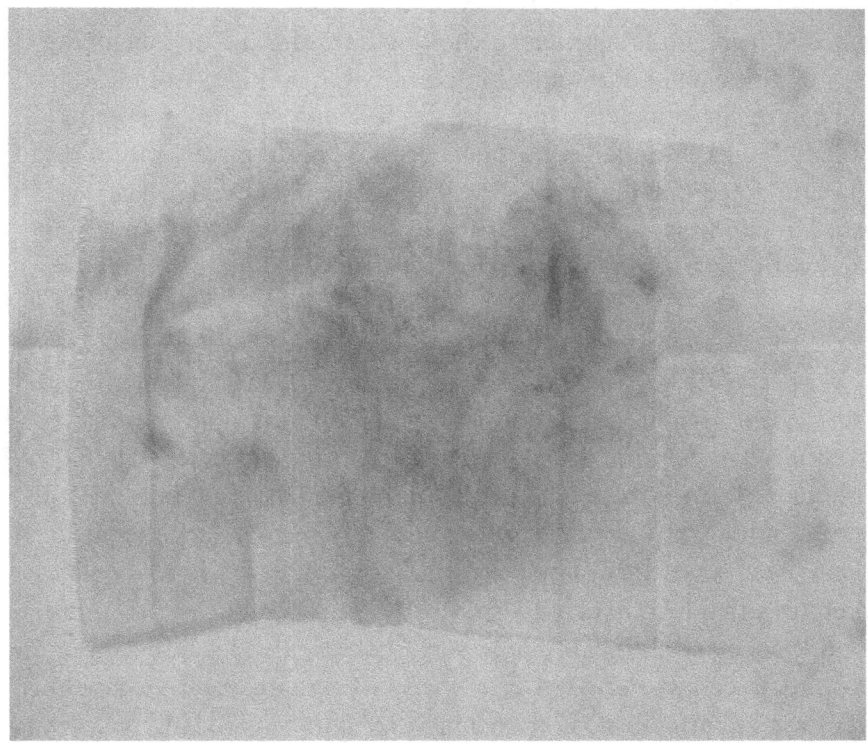

Figure 1. A wipe taken from employee's hands turned red, indicating the presence of lead.

Cabinets had multiple full containers of unleaded gasoline for the fuel truck and the golf cart. None of the cabinets were labeled. Fifty-five gallon drums were stored against the outside wall of the hangar. Some of the labels on these drums were illegible or missing. We observed open containers of used engine oil stored in buckets on the hangar floor.

We observed a layer of dust throughout the hangar and office areas. The owners reported that they performed the housekeeping themselves when they could. They reported using a leaf blower and a kitchen degreaser to clean the hangar floor. Compressed air was occasionally used to remove dust. Small parts, tools, and metal shavings were present on and around the workbench area, desktops, and open shelving units. Employees wore the same clothes and shoes from work to home where the contaminated clothing was laundered.

Aircraft idling in front of or moving past the hangar were loud. This noise was generated by the flight school's aircraft and by aircraft arriving or departing from the facilities on either side of the hangar. Flight instructors and students inside the cockpit wore earmuffs for hearing protection that also facilitated in-flight communication. Those working in the hangar did not routinely wear hearing protection but reported wearing ear plugs when grinding metal parts or when starting aircraft engines during a repair.

We observed that a child had full access to most areas in the hangar. His toys were present in the aircraft maintenance area. Twice we observed the child putting metal objects from the hangar floor into his mouth. The father quickly retrieved these objects. Children present in the hangar may be exposed to lead and other metals, choking hazards, and oils, machine fluids, and metal shavings. Cognitive and neurological impairment in children from lead exposure is irreversible and can result in lowered intelligence, learning impairment, and behavior problems. CDC recently lowered the level of concern for children from 10 µg/dL to a reference level of 5 µg/dL and noted that evidence shows impairment at even lower levels [CDC 2012a]. Lead exposure in children occurs primarily via ingestion when they put their hands or items contaminated with lead dust into their mouths.

An EPA representative used an x-ray fluorescence analyzer to test for lead at the child's residence on the same day we performed our evaluation. She reported lead paint on all four sides of the house exterior, on the sunroom window trim, and on the front door inside the house. In addition, three pieces of ceramic dinnerware tested positive at more than 5.0 milligrams per square centimeter. She observed lead paint chipping and flaking into the soil around the house. She also tested the tap water at the workplace and the residence for lead. The concentration at the workplace was 0.015 parts per million (ppm); in the residence it was 0.009 ppm. The EPA requires that lead in drinking water systems be below 0.015 ppm. One seat in a plane at the workplace and the seat of a personal vehicle also tested positive for lead at > 1.0 milligrams per square centimeter [EPA 2012]. The EPA representative gave the parents recommendations for remediating these non-occupational sources of lead.

Conclusions

Airborne lead exposures were below occupational exposure limits in the workplace. Employees had blood lead levels below 10 µg/dL and were asymptomatic. Surface contamination with lead was found in several work areas, and certain job activities, including sandblasting spark plugs and cleaning, were noted to have a higher risk for lead exposure. Recommendations were made to control exposures and to exclude children from the workplace.

Recommendations

On the basis of our findings, we recommend the actions listed below. These recommendations apply to the owners and employees, not children, who should not be allowed in the hangar. Our recommendations are based on an approach known as the hierarchy of controls (Appendix: Occupational Exposure Limits and Health Effects). This approach groups actions by their likely effectiveness in reducing or removing hazards. In most cases, the preferred approach is to eliminate hazardous materials or processes and install engineering controls to reduce exposure or shield employees. Until such controls are in place, or if they are not effective or feasible, administrative measures and personal protective equipment may be needed.

Elimination and Substitution

Eliminating or substituting hazardous processes or materials reduces hazards and protects employees more effectively than other approaches. Prevention through design, considering elimination or substitution when designing or developing a project, reduces the need for additional controls in the future. We recognize that this method of hazard reduction is not possible at this time. Alternatives to the leaded aviation fuel used at this facility are not available.

Engineering Controls

Engineering controls reduce employees' exposures by removing the hazard from the process or by placing a barrier between the hazard and the employee. Engineering controls protect employees effectively without placing primary responsibility of implementation on the employee.

1. Sandblast spark plugs outside the cabinet where they are stored. Install a local exhaust ventilation system for this activity that exhausts potentially contaminated air directly outdoors and away from the employee's breathing zone.

Administrative Controls

The term "administrative controls" refers to employer-dictated work practices and policies to reduce or prevent hazardous exposures. Their effectiveness depends on employer commitment and employee acceptance. Regular monitoring and reinforcement are necessary to ensure that policies and procedures are followed consistently.

1. Use damp and wet mopping and dusting methods. Discontinue dry cleaning methods using brooms, compressed air, and leaf blowers. These methods can aerosolize lead and other contaminants in the dust, which can then be inhaled.

2. Clean hangar surfaces regularly using a high efficiency particulate air filtered vacuum. The filter prevents lead and other particulates in the dust from being aerosolized during cleaning. Keep the work bench and work areas clean and free of debris.

3. Clean the carpet in the office areas with a high efficiency particulate air filtered vacuum. Consider replacing the carpet with a hard surface to facilitate cleaning.

4. Create a changing area separate from the main hangar. It is important to provide separate clean and dirty changing areas to prevent cross-contamination of the uniforms and the clothing employees wear home.

5. Launder work clothing on site or use a uniform laundry service. Inform the laundry service of potential for lead contamination on the uniforms.

6. Wear shoes worn only at the workplace or use disposable, slip-resistant booties over shoes when working in the facility and discard them right before leaving the workplace.

7. Prohibit eating and drinking in the facility. Move the refrigerator and food preparation devices into a separate dedicated eating area, and eat only in this area. Do not use a charcoal grill inside the facility.

8. Always wash hands thoroughly before eating and drinking, before and after glove use, and after the work shift. Do not wash hands with kerosene or other chemicals. Consider using hand wipe removal cloths to clean your hands. NIOSH research has shown that washing hands with soap and water is not completely effective in removing lead (and other toxic metals) from the skin. Consider purchasing lead removal wipes, either MEDTOX Scientific LeadTech Wipes™ or Hygenall Corporation Hygenall™.

9. Cover and label all containers of oil and other liquids.

10. Store and handle gasoline, solvents, and other flammable materials in a designated and approved flammable cabinet or storage room as required by OSHA [Code of Federal Regulations (CFR) 1910.106]. Cabinets must be appropriately labeled.

11. Do not allow children or their toys in the workplace.

12. Perform medical surveillance for lead according to the expert guidelines outlined in the appendix.

Personal Protective Equipment

Personal protective equipment is the least effective means for controlling hazardous exposures. Proper use of personal protective equipment requires a comprehensive program and a high level of employee involvement and commitment. The right personal protective equipment must be chosen for each hazard. Supporting programs such as training, change-out schedules, and medical assessment may be needed. Personal protective equipment should not be the sole method for controlling hazardous exposures. Rather, personal protective equipment should be used until effective engineering and administrative controls are in place.

1. Use a minimum of a NIOSH-approved N95 filtering facepiece respirator when sandblasting spark plugs until ventilation controls can be installed and monitoring shows that exposures are maintained below OELs.

2. Use respirators in the context of a program that meets the OSHA respiratory protection standard (29 CFR 1910.134). Among other things, this standard includes requirements for:
   a. Employees to be medically cleared by a physician to wear a respirator.
   b. Fit testing to ensure that proper seals are formed and maintained during routine movements and work tasks.
   c. Training on proper cleaning, storage, and maintenance of the respirator. For more information, refer to the OSHA guide for small businesses on respiratory protection, which can be found at http://www.osha.gov/Publications/3384small-entity-for-respiratory-protection-standard-rev.pdf. Additional information on respirators is available at http://www.cdc.gov/niosh/topics/respirators/.

3. Use a minimum of a NIOSH-approved N-95 filtering facepiece respirator when cleaning dusty areas.

4. Use nitrile rubber, polyurethane, chlorinated polyethylene, or Viton gloves, as recommended by the manufacturer, when handling parts contaminated with aviation gasoline or when cleaning up aviation gasoline spills.

5. Monitor noise exposures on days of normal and high aircraft traffic. Wear ear plugs when aircraft engines are started and when aircraft are idling near the hangar. If noise levels exceed the OSHA action level (AL), establish a hearing conservation program according to 29 CFR 1910.125. Also note that lead can damage the nerves responsible for hearing. Additionally, lead and noise have a synergistic effect, meaning that simultaneous exposure to both agents can cause more hearing loss than the effect of exposure to each of these separately.

Appendix: Occupational Exposure Limits and Health Effects

NIOSH investigators refer to mandatory (legally enforceable) and recommended OELs for chemical, physical, and biological agents when evaluating workplace hazards. OELs have been developed by federal agencies and safety and health organizations to prevent adverse health effects from workplace exposures. Generally, OELs suggest levels of exposure that most employees may be exposed to for up to 10 hours per day, 40 hours per week, for a working lifetime, without experiencing adverse health effects. However, not all employees will be protected if their exposures are maintained below these levels. Some may have adverse health effects because of individual susceptibility, a pre-existing medical condition, or a hypersensitivity (allergy). In addition, some hazardous substances act in combination with other exposures, with the general environment, or with medications or personal habits of the employee to produce adverse health effects. Most OELs address airborne exposures, but some substances can be absorbed directly through the skin and mucous membranes.

Most OELs are expressed as a TWA exposure. A TWA refers to the average exposure during a normal 8- to 10-hour workday. Some chemical substances and physical agents have recommended short-term exposure limit (STEL) or ceiling values. Unless otherwise noted, the STEL is a 15-minute TWA exposure. It should not be exceeded at any time during a workday. The ceiling limit should not be exceeded at any time.

In the United States, OELs have been established by federal agencies, professional organizations, state and local governments, and other entities. Some OELs are legally enforceable limits; others are recommendations.

- The U.S. Department of Labor OSHA PELs (29 CFR 1910 [general industry]; 29 CFR 1926 [construction industry]; and 29 CFR 1917 [maritime industry]) are legal limits. These limits are enforceable in workplaces covered under the Occupational Safety and Health Act of 1970.

- NIOSH RELs are recommendations based on a critical review of the scientific and technical information and the adequacy of methods to identify and control the hazard. NIOSH RELs are published in the *NIOSH Pocket Guide to Chemical Hazards* [NIOSH 2010]. NIOSH also recommends risk management practices (e.g., engineering controls, safe work practices, employee education/training, personal protective equipment, and exposure and medical monitoring) to minimize the risk of exposure and adverse health effects.

- Other OELs commonly used and cited in the United States include the TLVs, which are recommended by ACGIH, a professional organization, and the workplace environmental exposure levels (WEELs), which are recommended by the American Industrial Hygiene Association, another professional organization. The TLVs and WEELs are developed by committee members of these associations from a review of the published, peer-reviewed literature. These OELs are not consensus standards. TLVs are considered voluntary exposure guidelines for use by industrial hygienists and others trained in this discipline "to assist in the control of health hazards" [ACGIH 2013]. WEELs have been established for some chemicals "when no other legal or authoritative limits exist" [AIHA 2011].

Outside the United States, OELs have been established by various agencies and organizations and include legal and recommended limits. The Institut für Arbeitsschutz der Deutschen Gesetzlichen Unfallversicherung (Institute for Occupational Safety and Health of the German Social Accident Insurance) maintains a database of international OELs from European Union member states, Canada (Québec), Japan, Switzerland, and the United States. The database, available at http://www.dguv.de/ifa/en/gestis/limit_values/index.jsp, contains international limits for more than 1,500 hazardous substances and is updated periodically.

OSHA requires an employer to furnish employees a place of employment free from recognized hazards that cause or are likely to cause death or serious physical harm [Occupational Safety and Health Act of 1970 (Public Law 91–596, sec. 5(a)(1))]. This is true in the absence of a specific OEL. It also is important to keep in mind that OELs may not reflect current health-based information.

When multiple OELs exist for a substance or agent, NIOSH investigators generally encourage employers to use the lowest OEL when making risk assessment and risk management decisions. NIOSH investigators also encourage use of the hierarchy of controls approach to eliminate or minimize workplace hazards. This includes, in order of preference, the use of (1) substitution or elimination of the hazardous agent, (2) engineering controls (e.g., local exhaust ventilation, process enclosure, dilution ventilation), (3) administrative controls (e.g., limiting time of exposure, employee training, work practice changes, medical surveillance), and (4) personal protective equipment (e.g., respiratory protection, gloves, eye protection, hearing protection). Control banding, a qualitative risk assessment and risk management tool, is a complementary approach to protecting employee health. Control banding focuses on how broad categories of risk should be managed. Information on control banding is available at http://www.cdc.gov/niosh/topics/ctrlbanding/. This approach can be applied in situations where OELs have not been established or can be used to supplement existing OELs.

Below we provide the OELs and surface contamination limits for the compounds we measured, as well as a discussion of the potential health effects from exposure to these compounds.

Lead

Occupational exposure to inorganic lead occurs via inhalation of lead-containing dust and fume. In cases where careful attention to hygiene (for example, hand washing) is not practiced, smoking cigarettes or eating may represent another route of exposure among workers who handle lead and then transfer it to their mouth via contaminated hands.

Acute poisoning from inorganic lead rarely occurs today. Symptoms of chronic inorganic lead poisoning in adults may include headache, joint and muscle aches, weakness, fatigue, irritability, depression, constipation, anorexia, and abdominal discomfort [Moline and Landrigan 2005].

Lead can affect every body system. At levels over 40 μg/dL, infertility and reduced sex drive is seen in both genders and males may experience impotence. Lead can cause damage to organs even at lower levels. For example, kidney damage may be seen with blood lead levels under 20 μg/dL and anemia may occur with blood lead levels under 10 μg/dL [ATSDR 2007].

In most cases, an individual's blood lead level is a good indication of recent exposure to lead because its half-life (the time it takes for the quantity in the body to be reduced by half its initial value) is 1–2 months [Lauwerys and Hoet 2001; Moline and Landrigan 2005; NCEH 2005]. Most lead in the body is stored in the bones, with a half-life of years to decades. Bone lead can be measured using K-shell x-ray fluorescence instruments, but these are primarily research based and are not widely available. Elevated zinc protoporphyrin levels have also been used as an indicator of chronic lead intoxication; however, other factors, such as iron deficiency, can cause an elevated zinc protoporphyrin level, so monitoring the BLL over time is more specific for evaluating chronic occupational lead exposure.

The National Toxicology Program recently released a monograph on the health effects of low-level lead [National Toxicology Program 2012]. In adults, the National Toxicology Program found sufficient evidence that BLLs < 5 μg/dL are associated with decreased renal function, and that maternal BLLs < 5 μg/dL are associated with reduced fetal growth. There is limited evidence that BLLs < 5 μg/dL are associated with essential tremor. There is sufficient evidence that BLLs < 10 μg/dL are associated with increased blood pressure, hypertension, and essential tremor, and that maternal BLLs < 10 μg/dL are associated with increased spontaneous abortion and preterm birth. There is limited evidence that BLLs < 10 μg/dL are associated with increased cardiovascular mortality, decreased auditory function, amyotrophic lateral sclerosis, and decreased cognitive function. Inorganic lead is reasonably anticipated to cause cancer in humans [ATSDR 2007].

A panel of experts published guidelines for preventing acute and chronic effects of adult lead poisoning [Kosnett et al. 2007]. They recommended removing an employee from exposure if a single BLL exceeds 30 μg/dL, or if two measurements taken over 4 weeks exceed 20 μg/dL. Removal should be considered if control measures over an extended period do not decrease BLLs to < 10 μg/dL. The panel also recommended quarterly BLL testing if the BLL is 10–19 μg/dL and semiannual testing if the BLL is < 10 μg/dL. Pregnant women should avoid BLLs > 5 μg/dL. The California Department of Public Health and the Council of State and Territorial Epidemiologists endorsed these guidelines in 2009 [CSTE 2009].

OELs for inorganic lead may prevent overt symptoms of lead poisoning, but they are not sufficient to protect workers from more subtle adverse health effects like hypertension, renal dysfunction, and reproductive and cognitive effects [Schwartz and Hu 2007; Schwartz and Stewart 2007; Brown-Williams et al. 2009]. The OSHA general industry lead standard (29 CFR 1910.1025) includes elemental lead, all inorganic lead compounds, and a class of organic lead compounds called lead soaps and does not apply to other organic lead compounds. Under this standard, the PEL for airborne exposure is 50 $\mu g/m^3$ for an 8-hour TWA. The standard requires lowering the PEL for shifts exceeding 8 hours, medical monitoring for employees exposed to airborne lead at or above the AL of 30 $\mu g/m^3$ (8-hour TWA), medical removal of employees whose average BLL is 50 $\mu g/dL$ or greater, and economic protection for medically removed workers. Medically removed workers cannot return to jobs involving lead exposure until their BLL is below 40 $\mu g/dL$. NIOSH has an REL for lead of 50 $\mu g/m^3$ averaged over an 8-hour work shift [NIOSH 2012]. ACGIH has a TLV for lead of 50 $\mu g/m^3$ (8-hour TWA), with worker BLLs to be controlled to or below 30 $\mu g/dL$ and designation of lead as an animal carcinogen [ACGIH 2013].

TEL is not covered by the OSHA lead standard. The OSHA PEL and NIOSH REL for TEL is 75 $\mu g/m^3$, and the ACGIH TLV is 100 $\mu g/m^3$.

In homes with a family member occupationally exposed to lead, care must be taken to prevent "take home" of lead, that is, lead carried into the home on clothing, skin, hair, and in vehicles. Lead-contaminated surface dust represents a potential source of lead exposure, particularly for young children. This may occur either by direct hand-to-mouth contact, or indirectly from hand-to-mouth contact with contaminated clothing, cigarettes, or food. Studies have found a significant correlation between resident children's BLLs and house dust lead levels [Farfel and Chisholm 1990]. High BLLs in resident children and elevated concentrations of lead in house dust have been found in the homes of workers employed in industries associated with high lead exposure [Grandjean and Bach 1986]. Particular effort should be made to ensure that children of persons who work in these high lead exposure industries receive a BLL test. The current CDC screening guidelines for children use 5 $\mu g/dL$ as a "reference level" in order to intervene and prevent long-term cognitive deficits. Irreversible cognitive function deficits can occur at levels even lower than 5 $\mu g/dL$ [CDC 2012b].

In the workplace, generally there is little or no correlation between surface lead levels and employee exposures because ingestion exposures are highly dependent on personal hygiene practices and available facilities for maintaining personal hygiene. No current federal standard provides a permissible limit for lead contamination of surfaces in occupational settings.

References

ACGIH [2013]. 2013 TLVs® and BEIs®: threshold limit values for chemical substances and physical agents and biological exposure indices. Cincinnati, OH: American Conference of Governmental Industrial Hygienists.

AIHA [2011]. AIHA 2011 Emergency response planning guidelines (ERPG) & workplace environmental exposure levels (WEEL) handbook. Fairfax, VA: American Industrial Hygiene Association.

ATSDR [2007]. Toxicological profile for lead. Atlanta, GA: U.S. Department of Health and Human Services. Agency for Toxic Substances and Disease Registry.

Brown-Williams H, Lichterman J, Kosnett M [2009]. Indecent exposure: lead puts workers and families at risk. Health Research in Action, University of California, Berkeley. Perspectives *4*(1):1–9.

CDC (Centers for Disease Control and Prevention) [1991]. Preventing lead poisoning in young children. [http://www.cdc.gov/nceh/lead/publications/books/plpyc/contents.htm]. Date accessed: July 2013.

CDC (Centers for Disease Control and Prevention) [2009]. CDC lead prevention tips. [http://www.cdc.gov/nceh/lead/tips.htm]. Date accessed: July 2013.

CDC (Centers for Disease Control and Prevention) [2011]. Adult blood lead epidemiology and surveillance --- United States, 2008--2009. MMWR 60(25):841–845. [http://www.cdc.gov/mmwr/preview/mmwrhtml/mm6025a2.htm?s_cid=mm6025a2_w]. Date accessed: July 2013.

CDC (Centers for Disease Control and Prevention) [2012a]. Announcement: response to the advisory committee on childhood lead poisoning prevention report, low level lead exposure harms children: a renewed call for primary prevention. MMWR *61*(20):383. [http://www.cdc.gov/mmwr/preview/mmwrhtml/mm6120a6.htm?s_cid=mm6120a6_e%0d%0a]. Date accessed: July 2013.

CDC (Centers for Disease Control and Prevention) [2012b]. Blood lead levels in children. [http://www.cdc.gov/nceh/lead/ACCLPP/Lead_Levels_in_Children_Fact_Sheet.pdf]. Date accessed: July 2013.

CFR. Code of Federal Regulations. Washington, DC: U.S. Government Printing Office, Office of the Federal Register.

CSTE [2009]. Public health reporting and national notification for elevated blood lead levels. CSTE position statement 09-OH-02. Atlanta: CSTE 2009. [http://c.ymcdn.com/sites/www.cste.org/resource/resmgr/PS/09-OH-02.pdf]. Date accessed: July 2013.

EPA [2008]. Lead emissions from the use of leaded aviation gasoline in the United States – technical support document. United States Environmental Protection Agency. EPA420-R-08-020. Published October 2008.

EPA [2010]. Regulatory announcement: advance notice of proposed rulemaking on lead emissions from piston-engine aircraft using leaded aviation gasoline. EPA Office of Transportation and Air Quality. Publication number EPA-420-F-10-013. April 2010.

EPA [2012]. Pueblo lead testing. Golden, Colorado: United States Environmental Protection Agency, Region 8.

Farfel MR, Chisholm JJ [1990]. Health and environmental outcomes of traditional and modified practices for abatement of residential lead–based paint. Am J Pub Health $80(10):1240–1245$.

Grandjean P, Bach E [1986]. Indirect exposures: the significance of bystanders at work and at home. Am Ind Hyg Assoc J $47(12):819–824$.

Lauwerys RR, Hoet P [2001]. Biological monitoring of exposure to inorganic and organometallic substances. In: Industrial chemical exposure: guidelines for biological monitoring. 3rd ed. Boca Raton, FL: CRC Press, LLC, pp. 21–180.

Kosnett MJ, Wedeen RP, Rothenberg SJ, Hipkins KL, Materna BL, Schwartz BS, Hu H, Woolf A [2007]. Recommendations for medical management of adult blood lead exposure. Environ Health Perspect $115(3):463–471$.

Miranda ML, Anthopolos R, Hastings D [2011]. A geospatial analysis of the effects of aviation gasoline on childhood blood lead levels. Environ Health Perspect $119(10):1513–1516$.

Moline JM, Landrigan PJ [2005]. Lead. In: Rosenstock L, Cullen MR, Brodkin CA, Redlich CA, eds. Textbook of clinical occupational and environmental medicine. 2nd ed. Philadelphia, PA: Elsevier Saunders, pp. 967–979.

NCEH [2005]. Third national report on human exposure to environmental chemicals. Atlanta, GA: U.S. Department of Health and Human Services, Centers for Disease Control and Prevention. National Center for Environmental Health Publication number 05–0570.

NIOSH [2010]. NIOSH pocket guide to chemical hazards. Cincinnati, OH: U.S. Department of Health and Human Services, Centers for Disease Control and Prevention, National Institute for Occupational Safety and Health, DHHS (NIOSH) Publication No. 2012-168c. [http://www.cdc.gov/niosh/npg/]. Date accessed: July 2013.

NIOSH [2013]. NIOSH manual of analytical methods (NMAM®), 4th ed. Schlecht PC, O'Connor PF, eds. Cincinnati, OH: U.S. Department of Health and Human Services, Centers for Disease Control and Prevention, National Institute for Occupational Safety and Health, DHHS (NIOSH) Publication 94–113 (August, 1994); 1st Supplement Publication 96–135, 2nd Supplement Publication 98–119; 3rd Supplement 2003–154. [http://www.cdc.gov/niosh/nmam/]. Date accessed: July 2013.

National Toxicology Program [2012]. Monograph on the health effects of low-level lead. Research Triangle Park, NC: U.S. Department of Health and Human Services, National Institutes of Health, National Institute of Environmental Health Sciences. [http://ntp.niehs.nih.gov/NTP/ohat/Lead/Final/MonographHealthEffectsLowLevelLead_prepublication_508.pdf]. Date accessed: July 2013.

Schwartz BS, Hu H [2007]. Adult lead exposure: time for change. Environ Health Perspect *115*(3):451–454.

Schwartz BS, Stewart WF [2007]. Lead and cognitive function in adults: a question and answers approach to a review of the evidence for cause, treatment, and prevention. Int Rev Psychiatry *19*(6):671–692.

Tenenbein M [1997]. Leaded gasoline abuse: the role of tetraethyl lead. Hum Exp Toxicol *16*(4):217–222.

Keywords: North American Industry Classification System 611512 (Aviation schools), lead, tetraethyl lead, TEL, organic lead, aviation school, airplane mechanic, blood lead levels

The Health Hazard Evaluation Program investigates possible health hazards in the workplace under the authority of Section 20(a)(6) of the Occupational Safety and Health Act of 1970, 29 U.S.C. 669(a)(6). The Health Hazard Evaluation Program also provides, upon request, technical assistance to federal, state, and local agencies to control occupational health hazards and to prevent occupational illness and disease. Regulations guiding the Program can be found in Title 42, Code of Federal Regulations, Part 85; Requests for Health Hazard Evaluations (42 CFR 85).

Acknowledgments

Analytical Support: Bureau Veritas North America and Pacific Toxicology Laboratories
Desktop Publisher: Mary Winfree
Editor: Ellen Galloway
Health Communicator: Stefanie Brown
Industrial Hygiene Field Assistance: Donald Booher, Karl Feldmann, and Teri Bayrich, EPA Region 8
Logistics: Donnie Booher and Karl Feldmann
Medical Field Assistance: Deborah Sammons

Availability of Report